I0209894

# 86 Bad Breath Meal and Juice Solutions:

## Eliminate Bad Breath and Dry Mouth Conditions Quickly and Permanently

By

**Joe Correa CSN**

# COPYRIGHT

© 2017 Live Stronger Faster Inc.

All rights reserved

Reproduction or translation of any part of this work beyond that permitted by section 107 or 108 of the 1976 United States Copyright Act without the permission of the copyright owner is unlawful.

This publication is designed to provide accurate and authoritative information in regard to the subject matter covered. It is sold with the understanding that neither the author nor the publisher is engaged in rendering medical advice. If medical advice or assistance is needed, consult with a doctor. This book is considered a guide and should not be used in any way detrimental to your health. Consult with a physician before starting this nutritional plan to make sure it's right for you.

# ACKNOWLEDGEMENTS

This book is dedicated to my friends and family that have had mild or serious illnesses so that you may find a solution and make the necessary changes in your life.

# 86 Bad Breath Meal and Juice Solutions:

## Eliminate Bad Breath and Dry Mouth Conditions Quickly and Permanently

By

**Joe Correa CSN**

# CONTENTS

Copyright

Acknowledgements

About The Author

Introduction

86 Bad Breath Meal and Juice Solutions: Eliminate Bad Breath and Dry Mouth Conditions Quickly and Permanently

Additional Titles from This Author

## ABOUT THE AUTHOR

After years of Research, I honestly believe in the positive effects that proper nutrition can have over the body and mind. My knowledge and experience has helped me live healthier throughout the years and which I have shared with family and friends. The more you know about eating and drinking healthier, the sooner you will want to change your life and eating habits.

Nutrition is a key part in the process of being healthy and living longer so get started today. The first step is the most important and the most significant.

# INTRODUCTION

86 Bad Breath Meal and Juice Solutions: Eliminate Bad Breath and Dry Mouth Conditions Quickly and Permanently

By Joe Correa CSN

The key to a healthy and clean digestive tract and fresh breath lies in the food we eat. Just like with everything else in our body, food has the ability to do some serious damage as well as the ability to heal us.

When we talk about bad breath, there are some specific foods we have to consume in order to clean our mouth and destroy the bacteria responsible for these problems. Apples, carrots, and celery are among the best foods to help you fight bad breath. Unsweetened black or green tea are also proven to help fight off bad breath. They contain some powerful antioxidants that help destroy the bacteria growing in your mouth and other parts of a digestive system. Parsley, ginger, and basil, on the other hand, have the ability to directly neutralize the effects of a heavy, garlic-based lunch. Some other, bad breath fighting foods are cherries, lettuce, and spinach.

These meal and juice recipes are based on the ingredients mentioned above and then combined with some other foods for a unique taste you will absolutely love. Make the decision to eliminate bad breath by using these recipes and start enjoying close-up encounters!

# 86 BAD BREATH MEAL AND JUICE SOLUTIONS: ELIMINATE BAD BREATH AND DRY MOUTH CONDITIONS QUICKLY AND PERMANENTLY

## JUICES

### 1.	Blueberry Lemon Juice

**Ingredients:**

1 cup of blueberries

1 whole lemon, halved

1 Golden Delicious apple, cored

1 whole kiwi, peeled and chopped

¼ tsp of ginger, ground

1 oz of water

**Preparation:**

Place the blueberries in a colander. Rinse well under cold running water and drain. Fill the measuring cup and reserve the rest in the refrigerator.

Peel the lemon and cut lengthwise in half. Set aside.

Wash the apple and cut lengthwise in half. Remove the core and cut into bite-sized pieces and set aside.

Peel the kiwi and cut into small pieces. Make sure to reserve the kiwi juice while cutting.

Now, combine blueberries, lemon, apple, and kiwi in a juicer and process until juiced. Transfer to a serving glass and stir in the ginger, water, and reserved kiwi juice.

Add some crushed ice and serve immediately.

**Nutrition information per serving:** Kcal: 217, Protein: 3.2g, Carbs: 66.2g, Fats: 1.3g

## 2.    Raspberry Lime Juice

**Ingredients:**

1 cup of raspberries

1 whole lime, peeled

1 medium-sized Red Delicious apple, cored

1 whole plum, pitted and chopped

1 oz of water

**Preparation:**

Place the raspberries in a colander and rinse well under cold running water. Drain and fill the measuring cup. Reserve the rest in the refrigerator. Set aside.

Peel the lime and cut lengthwise in half. Cut into quarters and set aside.

Wash the apple and cut lengthwise in half. Remove the core and cut into bite-sized pieces. Set aside.

Wash the plum and cut in half. Remove the pit and chop into small pieces. Set aside.

Now, combine raspberries, lime, apple, and plum in a juicer and process until juiced. Transfer to a serving glass and stir in the water.

Refrigerate for 10 minutes before serving.

**Nutrition information per serving:** Kcal: 173, Protein: 2.7g, Carbs: 55.7g, Fats: 1.4g

## 3.    Broccoli Fennel Juice

**Ingredients:**

2 cups of broccoli, chopped

1 cup of fennel, chopped

1 medium-sized Granny Smith's apple, cored

1 cup of fresh basil, chopped

1 oz of water

**Preparation:**

Wash the broccoli and trim off the outer leaves. Chop into small pieces and fill the measuring cup. Reserve the rest for later. Set aside.

Trim off the fennel stalks and outer wilted layers. Wash and chop the fennel into bite-sized pieces. Fill the measuring cup and reserve the rest for later. Set aside.

Wash the apple and cut lengthwise in half. Remove the core and chop into small pieces. Set aside.

Rinse the basil thoroughly under cold running water. Drain and torn into small pieces. Set aside.

Now, combine broccoli, fennel, apple, and basil in a juicer and process until juiced. Transfer to a serving glass and stir in the water.

Refrigerate for 10 minutes before serving.

**Nutrition information per serving:** Kcal: 140, Protein: 7.7g, Carbs: 41.8g, Fats: 1.3g

## 4. Cantaloupe Orange Juice

**Ingredients:**

1 cup of cantaloupe, chopped

1 large orange, peeled

1 cup of fresh mint, torn

1 cup of blackberries

¼ tsp of cinnamon, ground

**Preparation:**

Cut the cantaloupe in half. Scrape out the seeds and cut one large wedge. Peel and chop into small pieces. Fill the measuring cup and wrap the rest in a plastic foil. Refrigerate for later.

Peel the orange and divide into wedges. Cut each wedge in half and set aside.

Rinse the mint under cold running water and drain. Torn into small pieces and set aside.

Place the blackberries in a colander and rinse well. Drain and set aside.

Now, combine cantaloupe, orange, mint, and blackberries in a juicer and process until juiced. Transfer to a serving glass and stir in the cinnamon.

Add some ice and serve immediately.

**Nutrition information per serving:** Kcal: 157, Protein: 5.9g, Carbs: 51.9g, Fats: 1.5g

## 5. Pumpkin Lemon Juice

**Ingredients:**

1 cup of pumpkin, cubed

1 small Golden Delicious apple, cored and chopped

1 whole lemon, peeled and halved

1 large carrot, sliced

1 cup of watercress, torn

**Preparation:**

Cut the top of a pumpkin. Cut lengthwise in half and then scrape out the seeds. Cut one large wedge and peel it. Cut into small cubes and fill the measuring cup. Reserve the rest in the refrigerator.

Wash the apple and cut lengthwise in half. Remove the core and cut into bite-sized pieces. Set aside.

Peel the lemon and cut lengthwise in half. Set aside.

Wash and peel the carrot. Cut into thin slices and set aside.

Rinse the watercress thoroughly under cold running water. Drain and torn into small pieces. Set aside.

Now, combine pumpkin, apple, lemon, carrot, and watercress in a juicer and process until juiced. Transfer to a serving glass and add some ice before serving.

Enjoy!

**Nutrition information per serving:** Kcal: 126, Protein: 3.6g, Carbs: 37.8g, Fats: 0.7g

## 6.    Mango Strawberry Juice

**Ingredients:**

1 whole mango, chopped

1 cup of strawberries, chopped

1 whole lime, peeled

1 large pear, chopped

1 cup of fresh mint, torn

1 tbsp of coconut water

**Preparation:**

Peel the mango and chop into small chunks or cubes. Set aside.

Wash the strawberries and remove the stems. Cut into bite-sized pieces and fill the measuring cup. Reserve the rest in the refrigerator.

Peel the lime and cut lengthwise in half. Set aside.

Wash the pear and cut in half. Remove the core and chop into small pieces. Set aside.

Rinse the mint thoroughly under cold running water and drain. Torn into small pieces and set aside.

Now, combine mango, strawberries, lime, pear, and mint in a juicer and process until juiced. Transfer to serving glass and stir in the coconut water.

Add some crushed ice and serve immediately.

**Nutrition information per serving:** Kcal: 335, Protein: 5.7g, Carbs: 103g, Fats: 2.3g

## 7.    Grapefruit Apple Juice

**Ingredients:**

1 whole grapefruit, peeled and wedged

1 medium-sized apple, cored

3 whole apricots, pitted

1 cup of Swiss chard, torn

1 tbsp of liquid honey

¼ tsp of ginger, ground

**Preparation:**

Peel the grapefruit and divide into wedges. Cut each wedge in half and set aside.

Wash the apple and cut lengthwise in half. Remove the core and chop into bite-sized pieces. Set aside.

Wash the apricots and cut into halves. Chop all into small pieces and set aside.

Rinse the Swiss chard thoroughly under cold running water. Drain and torn into small pieces. Set aside.

Now, combine grapefruit, apple, apricots, and Swiss chard in a juicer and process until juiced. Transfer to a serving glass and stir in the honey and ginger.

Add few ice cubes and serve immediately.

**Nutrition information per serving:** Kcal: 212, Protein: 4.7g, Carbs: 61.9g, Fats: 1.1g

## 8. Cherry Pineapple Juice

**Ingredients:**

1 cup of cherries, pitted

1 cup of pineapple, chunked

1 cup of spinach, chopped

1 whole lemon, peeled

¼ tsp of cinnamon, ground

1 oz of water

**Preparation:**

Place the cherries in a medium colander. Rinse well under cold running water and remove the stems, if any. Cut each in half and remove the pits. Fill the measuring cup and reserve the rest in the refrigerator.

Using a sharp paring knife, cut the top of the pineapple. Gently remove all hard skin and slice it into thin slices. Fill the measuring cup and reserve the rest for later.

Rinse the spinach thoroughly under cold running water. Drain and chop into small pieces. Set aside.

Peel the lemon and cut lengthwise in half. Set aside.

Now, combine cherries, pineapple, spinach, and lemon in a juicer and process until juiced. Transfer to a serving glass and stir in the water.

Add some crushed ice and serve immediately.

**Nutrition information per serving:** Kcal: 196, Protein: 9.2g, Carbs: 59.3g, Fats: 1.5g

## 9. Tomato Parsley Juice

**Ingredients:**

2 medium-sized Roma tomatoes, chopped

1 cup of fresh parsley, torn

1 medium-sized artichoke, chopped

1 cup of Romaine lettuce, torn

¼ tsp of salt

¼ tsp of dried oregano, ground

**Preparation:**

Wash the tomatoes and place in a bowl. Chop into small pieces and make sure to reserve the tomato juice while cutting. Set aside.

Combine parsley and lettuce in a large colander. Rinse well under cold running water and drain. Torn into small pieces and set aside.

Wash the artichoke trim off the outer leaves. Chop into bite-sized pieces and fill the measuring cup. Reserve the rest in the refrigerator. Set aside.

Now, combine tomatoes, parsley, artichoke, and lettuce in a juicer and process until juiced. Transfer to a serving glass and stir in the salt and oregano.

Refrigerate for 10 minutes before serving.

Enjoy!

**Nutrition information per serving:** Kcal: 82, Protein: 8.7g, Carbs: 28.3g, Fats: 1.3g

## 10.    Avocado Beet Juice

**Ingredients:**

1 cup of avocado, cubed

1 cup of beets, sliced

1 cup of celery, cut into bite-sized pieces

1 whole lemon, peeled

1 oz of water

**Preparation:**

Peel the avocado and cut lengthwise in half. Remove the pit and cut into small cubes. Fill the measuring cup and reserve the rest in the refrigerator. Set aside.

Wash the beets and trim off the green ends. Slightly peel and cut into thin slices. Fill the measuring cup and reserve the rest for later.

Wash the celery and cut into bite-sized pieces. Fill the measuring cup and reserve the rest in the refrigerator.

Peel the lemon and cut lengthwise in half. Set aside.

Now, combine avocado, beets, celery, and lemon in a juicer. Process until juiced.

Transfer to a serving glass and stir in the water. Refrigerate for 10 minutes before serving.

**Nutrition information per serving:** Kcal: 264, Protein: 6.5g, Carbs: 34.2g, Fats: 22.5g

## 11. Papaya Orange Juice

**Ingredients:**

1 cup of papaya, chopped

1 large orange, peeled

1 small Granny Smith's apple, cored

1 cup of fresh mint, torn

1 tbsp of fresh basil, torn

**Preparation:**

Wash and peel the papaya. Cut lengthwise in half and scoop out the seeds. Cut into bite-sized pieces and fill the measuring cup. Reserve the rest in the refrigerator.

Peel the orange and divide into wedges. Cut each wedge in half and set aside.

Wash the apple and cut in half. Remove the core and cut into bite-sized pieces. Set aside.

Rinse the mint and basil thoroughly under cold running water. Drain and torn into small pieces. Set aside.

Now, combine papaya, orange, apple, mint, and basil in a juicer and process until juiced. Transfer to a serving glass and add some ice.

Serve immediately.

**Nutrition information per serving:** Kcal: 199, Protein: 4.1g, Carbs: 60.1g, Fats: 1.1g

## 12.   Cabbage Zucchini Juice

**Ingredients:**

1 cup of purple cabbage, torn

1 medium-sized zucchini, sliced

1 cup of celery, chopped

1 cup of cucumber, sliced

¼ tsp of ginger, ground

¼ tsp of turmeric, ground

¼ tsp of salt

**Preparation:**

Rinse the purple cabbage under cold running water. Drain and torn into small pieces and set aside.

Wash the zucchini and cut into thin slices. Set aside.

Wash the celery and chop into bite-sized pieces. Set aside.

Wash the cucumber and cut into slices. Fill the measuring cup and reserve the rest for later.

Now, combine cabbage, zucchini, celery, and cucumber in a juicer and process until juiced. Transfer to a serving glass and stir in the ginger, turmeric, and salt.

Refrigerate for 10 minutes before serving.

**Nutrition information per serving:** Kcal: 62, Protein: 4.7g, Carbs: 17.5g, Fats: 1g

## 13.    Strawberry Squash Juice

**Ingredients:**

1 cup of strawberries, chopped

1 cup of butternut squash, cubed

2 whole plums, pitted and chopped

1 medium-sized apple, cored

¼ tsp of ginger, ground

¼ tsp of turmeric, ground

**Preparation:**

Wash the strawberries and remove the stems. Cut into bite-sized pieces and fill the measuring cup. Reserve the rest in the refrigerator. Set aside.

Peel the butternut squash and cut lengthwise in half. Scoop out the seeds and wash the both halves. Cut into small cubes and fill the measuring cup. Wrap the rest of the squash in a plastic foil and refrigerate for later.

Wash the plums and cut in half. Remove the pits and cut into bite-sized pieces. Set aside.

Wash the apple and cut lengthwise in half. Remove the core and cut into bite-sized pieces. Set aside.

Now, combine strawberries, butternut squash, plum, and apple in a juicer and process until well juiced. Transfer to a serving glass and add some crushed ice.

Serve immediately.

**Nutrition information per serving:** Kcal: 214, Protein: 4.1g, Carbs: 65.2g, Fats: 1.2g

## 14.    Cauliflower Parsnip Juice

**Ingredients:**

1 cup of cauliflower, chopped

1 cup of parsnip, sliced

1 large carrot, sliced

1 cup of fennel, trimmed and chopped

1 whole lime, peeled

**Preparation:**

Wash the cauliflower and trim off the outer leaves. Cut into small pieces and fill the measuring cup. Reserve the rest for later.

Wash and peel the parsnip. Cut into thin slices and fill the measuring cup. Reserve the rest for later.

Trim off the fennel stalks and outer wilted layers. Wash and chop the fennel into bite-sized pieces. Fill the measuring cup and reserve the rest for later. Set aside.

Peel the lime and cut lengthwise in half. Set aside.

Now, combine cauliflower, parsnip, carrot, fennel, and lime in a juicer. Process until well juiced.

Transfer to a serving glass and refrigerate for 10 minutes before serving.

Add some turmeric or ginger for some extra taste. However, it's optional.

**Nutrition information per serving:** Kcal: 141, Protein: 5.6g, Carbs: 46.2g, Fats: 1.1g

## 15. Orange Pear Juice

**Ingredients:**

1 medium-sized orange, peeled

1 medium-sized pear, chopped

1 cup of beets, chopped

1 small Golden Delicious apple, chopped

¼ tsp of cinnamon, ground

¼ tsp of ginger, ground

**Preparation:**

Peel the orange and divide into wedges. Cut each wedge in half and set aside.

Wash the pear and cut in half. Remove the core and chop into small pieces. Set aside.

Wash the beets and trim off the green ends. Cut into slices and fill the measuring cup. Reserve the rest for later.

Wash the apple and cut lengthwise in half. Remove the core and cut into bite-sized pieces. Set aside.

Now, combine orange, pear, beets, and apple in a juicer and process until juiced.

Transfer to a serving glass and stir in the cinnamon and ginger. Add some ice before serving.

Enjoy!

**Nutrition information per serving:** Kcal: 234, Protein: 4.4g, Carbs: 73.1g, Fats: 0.8g

## 16.  Blueberry Grape Juice

**Ingredients:**

2 cups of blueberries

1 cup of black grapes

1 cup of fresh mint, torn

1 large banana, peeled

2 tbsp of milk

¼ tsp of cinnamon, ground

**Preparation:**

Place the blueberries in a colander. Rinse well under cold running water and drain. Set aside.

Wash the grapes and remove the stems. Fill the measuring cup and reserve the rest in the refrigerator. Set aside.

Wash the mint thoroughly under cold running water. Drain and torn into small pieces. Set aside.

Now, combine blueberries, grapes, mint, and banana in a juicer and process until juiced. Transfer to a serving glass and stir in the milk and cinnamon.

Refrigerate for 10 minutes before serving.

**Nutrition information per serving:** Kcal: 326, Protein: 6.2g, Carbs: 93.4g, Fats: 2.1g

## 17.    Crookneck Squash Juice

**Ingredients:**

1 cup of crookneck squash, cubed

1 large orange, peeled

1 large carrot, sliced

1 whole lemon, peeled

1 cup of cucumber, sliced

¼ tsp of turmeric, ground

**Preparation:**

Wash the squash and chop into small cubes. Fill the measuring cup and reserve the rest in the refrigerator. Set aside.

Peel the orange and divide into wedges. Cut each wedge in half and set aside.

Wash and peel the carrot. Cut into thin slices and set aside.

Peel the lemon and cut lengthwise in half. Set aside.

Wash the cucumber and cut into thin slices. Fill the measuring cup and reserve the rest for later.

Now, combine squash, orange, carrot, lemon, and cucumber in a juicer and process until juiced. Transfer to a serving glass and stir in the turmeric.

Add some crushed ice and serve immediately.

**Nutrition information per serving:** Kcal: 127, Protein: 4.6g, Carbs: 40.7g, Fats: 0.9g

## 18.    Kale Beet Juice

**Ingredients:**

1 cup of fresh kale, torn

1 cup of beets, sliced

1 small Granny Smith's apple, cored

1 cup of cantaloupe, cubed

¼ tsp of ginger, ground

**Preparation:**

Rinse the kale thoroughly under cold running water. Drain and torn into small pieces. Set aside.

Wash the beets and trim off the green ends. Cut into thin slices and fill the measuring cup. Reserve the rest for some other juice.

Wash the apple and cut lengthwise in half. Remove the core and cut into bite-sized pieces. Set aside.

Cut the cantaloupe in half. Scrape out the seeds and cut one large wedge. Peel and chop into small pieces. Fill the measuring cup and wrap the rest in a plastic foil. Refrigerate for later.

Now, combine kale, beets, apple, and cantaloupe in a juicer and process until juiced. Transfer to a serving glass and stir in the ginger.

Add some ice and serve immediately.

**Nutrition information per serving:** Kcal: 181, Protein: 7g, Carbs: 51.1g, Fats: 1.4g

## 19.    Kiwi Mint Juice

**Ingredients:**

2 whole kiwis, peeled

1 cup of fresh mint, torn

1 cup of cucumber, sliced

1 medium-sized Golden Delicious apple, cored

1 large banana, peeled

**Preparation:**

Peel the kiwis and cut lengthwise in half. Set aside.

Rinse the mint thoroughly under cold running water and drain. Torn into small pieces and set aside.

Wash the cucumber and cut into thin slices. Fill the measuring cup and reserve the rest for later. Set aside.

Wash the apple and cut lengthwise in half. Remove the core and cut into bite-sized pieces. Set aside.

Peel the banana and cut into thin slices. Set aside.

Now, combine kiwis, cucumber, apple, and banana in a juicer and process until juiced. Transfer to a serving glass and add some ice.

Serve immediately.

**Nutrition information per serving:** Kcal: 272, Protein: 4.8g, Carbs: 79.8g, Fats: 1.7g

## 20.   Blackberry Mango Juice

**Ingredients:**

1 cup of blackberries

1 cup of mango, chunked

3 whole apricots, chopped

1 cup of fresh spinach, torn

1 whole lime, peeled

**Preparation:**

Rinse the blackberries using a large colander. Drain and set aside.

Peel the mango and cut into small chunks. Fill the measuring cup and reserve the rest for later. Set aside.

Wash the apricots and cut in half. Remove the pits and chop into small pieces. Set aside.

Rinse the spinach thoroughly under cold running water. Drain and torn into small pieces. Set aside.

Peel the lime and cut lengthwise in half. Set aside.

Now, combine blackberries, mango, apricots, spinach, and lime in a juicer. Process until juiced. Transfer to a serving glass and refrigerate for 10 minutes before serving.

Enjoy!

**Nutrition information per serving:** Kcal: 201, Protein: 11.1g, Carbs: 61.5g, Fats: 2.6g

## 21.    Cranberry Peppermint Juice

**Ingredients:**

1 cup of cranberries

3 whole apricots, pitted and chopped

1 small Golden Delicious apple, cored

1 cup of cherries, pitted

1 tsp of peppermint extract

3 tbsp of coconut water

**Preparation:**

Rinse the cranberries using a large colander. Drain and set aside.

Wash the apricots and cut in half. Remove the pits and chop into small pieces. Set aside.

Wash the apple and cut lengthwise in half. Remove the core and chop into small pieces. Set aside.

Rinse the cherries under cold running water. Drain and cut each cherry in half. Remove the pits and set aside.

Now, combine cranberries, apricots, apple, and cherries in a juicer and process until juiced. Transfer to a serving glass and stir in the peppermint extract and coconut water.

Sprinkle with some finely chopped mint for some extra taste. However, it's optional.

Add few ice cubes and serve immediately.

**Nutrition information per serving:** Kcal: 216, Protein: 3.8g, Carbs: 66.1g, Fats: 1.1g

## 22.    Parsley Cucumber Juice

**Ingredients:**

2 cups of parsley, torn

1 whole cucumber, sliced

1 cup of celery, chopped

1 whole leek, chopped

1 cup of beet greens, torn

¼ tsp of turmeric powder, ground

¼ tsp of cumin, ground

**Preparation:**

Combine parsley and beet greens in a large colander. Rinse well under cold running water and drain. Torn into small pieces and set aside.

Wash the cucumber and cut into thin slices. Set aside.

Wash the celery and chop into small pieces. Fill the measuring cup and reserve the rest in the refrigerator. Set aside.

Wash the leek and chop into bite-sized pieces. Set aside.

Now, combine parsley, beet greens, cucumber, celery, and leek in a juicer and process until juiced. Transfer to a serving glass and stir in the turmeric and cumin.

Serve immediately.

**Nutrition information per serving:** Kcal: 127, Protein: 8.4g, Carbs: 35.7g, Fats: 1.7g

## 23.　Honeydew Melon-Swiss Chard Juice

### Ingredients:

1 large wedge of honeydew melon, peeled and cubed

1 cup of Swiss chard, torn

1 large carrot, peeled and sliced

1 cup of cucumber, sliced

1 small ginger knob, peeled

¼ tsp of turmeric, ground

2 oz of water

### Preparation:

Cut melon lengthwise in half. Scoop out the seeds and then wash. Cut one large wedge and peel it. Cut into small cubes and set aside.

Rinse the Swiss chard thoroughly under cold running water. Drain and torn into small pieces. Set aside.

Wash and peel the carrot. Cut into thin slices and set aside.

Wash the cucumber and cut into thin slices. Fill the measuring cup and reserve the rest for later. Set aside.

Peel the ginger knob and cut into small pieces. Set aside.

Now, combine melon, Swiss chard, carrot, and cucumber in a juicer and process until juiced. Transfer to a serving glass and stir in the turmeric and water.

Refrigerate for 10 minutes before serving.

**Nutrition information per serving:** Kcal: 92, Protein: 2.6g, Carbs: 25.7g, Fats: 0.5g

## 24. Celery Apple Juice

**Ingredients:**

1 cup of celery, chopped

1 large Granny Smith's apple, cored and chopped

1 small ginger knob, peeled

1 cup of fresh mint, torn

¼ tsp of liquid honey

1 oz of water

**Preparation:**

Wash the celery and chop into small pieces. Fill the measuring cup and reserve the rest for later.

Wash the apple and cut lengthwise in half. Remove the core and cut into bite-sized pieces. Set aside.

Peel the ginger knob and chop into small pieces. Set aside.

Rinse the mint thoroughly under cold running water. Dran and torn into small pieces.

Now, combine celery, apple, ginger, and mint in a juicer and process until well juiced. Transfer to a serving glass and stir in the honey and water.

Refrigerate for 10 minutes before serving.

Enjoy!

**Nutrition information per serving:** Kcal: 121, Protein: 2.6g, Carbs: 35.8g, Fats: 0.8g

## 25. Plum Pomegranate Juice

**Ingredients:**

3 whole plums, pitted and chopped

1 cup of pomegranate seeds

1 cup of pumpkin, cubed

1 medium-sized orange, peeled

¼ tsp of ginger, ground

1 oz of water

**Preparation:**

Wash the plums and cut into halves. Remove the pits and chop into small pieces. Set aside.

Cut the top of the pomegranate fruit using a sharp paring knife. Slice down to each of the white membranes inside of the fruit. Pop the seeds into a measuring cup and set aside.

Cut the top of a pumpkin. Cut lengthwise in half and then scrape out the seeds. Cut one large wedge and peel it. Cut into small cubes and fill the measuring cup. Reserve the rest in the refrigerator.

Peel the orange and divide into wedges. Cut each wedge in half and set aside.

Now, combine plums, pomegranate, pumpkin, and orange in a juicer. Process until juiced. Transfer to a serving glass and stir in the ginger and water.

Refrigerate for 10 minutes before serving.

Enjoy!

**Nutrition information per serving:** Kcal: 214, Protein: 5.2g, Carbs: 61.8g, Fats: 1.8g

## 26.    Pepper Fennel Juice

**Ingredients:**

2 large red bell peppers, seeds removed

1 cup of fennel, trimmed and chopped

1 cup of spinach, torn

1 cup of cucumber, sliced

¼ tsp of salt

¼ tsp of cayenne pepper, ground

**Preparation:**

Wash the bell peppers and cut each lengthwise in half. Remove the stem and seeds. Chop into small pieces and set aside.

Trim off the fennel stalks and outer wilted layers. Wash and chop the fennel into bite-sized pieces. Fill the measuring cup and reserve the rest for later. Set aside.

Rinse the spinach thoroughly under cold running water. Drain and torn into small pieces. Fill the measuring cup and reserve the rest in the refrigerator.

Wash the cucumber and cut into thin slices. Fill the measuring cup and reserve the rest for later.

Now, combine bell peppers, fennel, spinach, and cucumber in a juicer and process until juiced. Transfer to a serving glass and stir in the salt and cayenne pepper.

Serve cold.

**Nutrition information per serving:** Kcal: 125, Protein: 10.6g, Carbs: 35.65g, Fats: 2.1g

## 27.    Peach Apple Juice

**Ingredients:**

1 large peach, pitted

1 medium-sized Granny Smith's apple, cored

1 whole lemon, peeled

1 cup of mango, chunked

¼ tsp of cinnamon, ground

**Preparation:**

Wash the peach and cut in half. Remove the pit and chop into small pieces. Set aside.

Wash the apple and cut lengthwise in half. Remove the core and chop into bite-sized pieces. Set aside.

Peel the lemon and cut lengthwise in half. Set aside.

Peel the mango and cut into small chunks. Fill the measuring cup and reserve the rest in the refrigerator. Set aside.

Now, combine peach, apple, lemon, and mango in a juicer and process until juiced. Transfer to a serving glass and stir in the cinnamon.

Add some crushed ice and serve immediately.

Enjoy!

**Nutrition information per serving:** Kcal: 236, Protein: 4.3g, Carbs: 69.5g, Fats: 1.5g

## 28.    Avocado Blueberry Juice

**Ingredients:**

1 cup of avocado, cubed

1 cup of blueberries

1 whole grapefruit, peeled

1 small Red Delicious apple, cored

1 tsp of peppermint extract

**Preparation:**

Peel the avocado and cut lengthwise in half. Remove the pit and cut into small cubes. Fill the measuring cup and reserve the rest in the refrigerator.

Place the blueberries in a colander. Rinse well under cold running water and drain. Set aside.

Peel the grapefruit and divide into wedges. Cut each wedge in half and set aside.

Wash the apple and cut lengthwise in half. Remove the core and cut into bite-sized pieces. Set aside.

Now, combine avocado, blueberries, grapefruit, and apple in a juicer and process until juiced. Transfer to a serving glass and stir in the peppermint extract. Refrigerate for 15 minutes before serving.

**Nutrition information per serving:** Kcal: 436, Protein: 6.4g, Carbs: 69.5g, Fats: 23.2g

## 29.  Strawberry Lemon Juice

**Ingredients:**

1 cup of strawberries, chopped

1 whole lemon, peeled

1 large banana, chunked

1 cup of pineapple, chunked

1 tbsp of fresh mint, finely chopped

**Preparation:**

Wash the strawberries and remove the stems. Chop into small pieces and fill the measuring cup. Reserve the rest in the refrigerator.

Peel the lemon and cut lengthwise in half. Set aside.

Peel the banana and cut into small chunks. Set aside.

Cut the top of the pineapple using a sharp paring knife. Gently remove all hard skin and slice it into thin slices. Fill the measuring cup and reserve the rest for later.

Now, combine strawberries, lemon, banana, and pineapple in a juicer. Process until juiced. Transfer to a serving glass and stir in the mint.

Add few ice cubes and serve immediately.

**Nutrition information per serving:** Kcal: 224, Protein: 4.1g, Carbs: 69.4g, Fats: 1.3g

## 30.    Watermelon Celery Juice

**Ingredients:**

1 cup of watermelon, diced

1 cup of celery, chopped

1 cup of cherries, pitted

1 small ginger knob, peeled

1 oz of water

¼ tsp of cinnamon, ground

**Preparation:**

Cut the watermelon in half. Cut one large wedge and wrap the rest in a plastic foil and refrigerate. Dice the wedge and remove the pits. Fill the measuring cup and set aside.

Wash the celery and cut into small pieces. Fill the measuring cup and reserve the rest for later. Set aside.

Rinse the cherries under cold running water using a colander. Drain and cut each in half. Remove the pits and set aside.

Peel the ginger knob and cut into small pieces. Set aside.

Now, combine watermelon, celery, cherries, and ginger knob in a juicer and process until juiced. Transfer to a serving glass and stir in the water and cinnamon. Add some ice and serve immediately.

**Nutrition information per serving:** Kcal: 143, Protein: 3.4g, Carbs: 40.2g, Fats: 0.7g

## 31.    Lettuce Tomato Juice

**Ingredients:**

2 cups of Romaine lettuce, chopped

1 medium-sized Roma tomato, chopped

1 cup of mustard greens, torn

1 cup of parsley, torn

1 whole cucumber, sliced

¼ tsp of turmeric, ground

¼ tsp of salt

**Preparation:**

Rinse the lettuce thoroughly under cold running water. Chop into small pieces and set aside.

Wash the tomato and place in a bowl. Chop into bite-sized pieces and reserve the tomato juice while cutting. Set aside.

Combine mustard greens and parsley in a large colander. Rinse well and drain. Torn into small pieces and set aside.

Wash the cucumber and cut into thin slices. Set aside.

Now, combine lettuce, tomato, mustard greens, parsley, and cucumber in a juicer and process until juiced. Transfer to a serving glass and stir in the turmeric, salt, and reserved tomato juice.

Refrigerate for 10 minutes before serving.

Enjoy!

**Nutrition information per serving:** Kcal: 85, Protein: 7.6g, Carbs: 25.3g, Fats: 1.6g

## 32.   Potato Artichoke Juice

**Ingredients:**

1 cup of sweet potatoes, cubed

1 medium-sized artichoke, chopped

1 small zucchini, sliced

1 whole lime, peeled

1 large carrot, sliced

¼ tsp of salt

¼ tsp of turmeric, ground

**Preparation:**

Peel the potatoes and cut into small cubes. Place in a deep pot and add 3 cups of water. Bring it to a boil and cook for 5 minutes. Remove from the heat and drain well. Set aside to cool completely.

Wash the artichoke and trim off the outer leaves. Cut into small pieces and fill the measuring cup. Reserve the rest in the refrigerator.

Peel the zucchini and cut into thin slices. Set aside.

Peel the lime and cut lengthwise in half. Set aside.

Wash and peel the carrot. Cut into thin slices and set aside.

Now, combine potatoes, artichoke, zucchini, lime, and carrots in a juicer and process until juiced. Transfer to a serving glass and stir in the salt and turmeric.

Refrigerate for 10 minutes before serving.

**Nutrition information per serving:** Kcal: 177, Protein: 8.6g, Carbs: 54.5g, Fats: 0.8g

## 33.    Cantaloupe Cranberry Juice

**Ingredients:**

1 cup of cantaloupe, diced

1 cup of cranberries

1 cup of blackberries

1 small Golden Delicious apple, cored

¼ tsp of cinnamon, ground

¼ tsp of ginger, ground

**Preparation:**

Cut the cantaloupe in half. Scrape out the seeds and cut one large wedge. Peel and dice into small pieces. Fill the measuring cup and wrap the rest in a plastic foil. Refrigerate for later.

Combine cranberries and blackberries in a large colander. Rinse well under cold running water and drain. Set aside.

Wash the apple cut lengthwise in half. Remove the core and cut into bite-sized pieces. Set aside.

Now, combine cantaloupe, cranberries, blackberries, and apple in a juicer and process until well juiced. Transfer to a serving glass and stir in the cinnamon and ginger.

Add some crushed ice and serve immediately.

Enjoy!

**Nutrition information per serving:** Kcal: 169, Protein: 4.1g, Carbs: 56.3g, Fats: 1.3g

## 34.    Apricot Honey Juice

**Ingredients:**

1 cup of apricots, pitted and halved

1 tbsp of liquid honey

1 small Granny Smith's apple, cored

1 small pear, chopped

1 whole lemon, peeled and halved

1 cup of fresh mint, torn

**Preparation:**

Wash the apricots and cut each lengthwise in half. Remove the pits and fill the measuring cup. Reserve the rest in the refrigerator for some other juice.

Wash the apple and cut lengthwise in half. Remove the core and chop into bite-sized pieces. Set aside.

Wash the pear and cut in half. Remove the core and cut into small pieces. Set aside.

Peel the lemon and cut lengthwise in half. Set aside.

Rinse the mint thoroughly under cold running water. Drain and torn into small pieces. Set aside.

Now, combine apricots, apple, pear, lemon, and mint in a juicer and process until well juiced. Transfer to a serving glass and add some ice before serving.

Enjoy!

**Nutrition information per serving:** Kcal: 217, Protein: 4.9g, Carbs: 68.5g, Fats: 1.5g

## 35.    Fennel Spinach Juice

**Ingredients:**

1 cup of fennel, chopped

1 cup of spinach, torn

1 cup of broccoli, chopped

1 whole lemon, peeled

1 whole lime, peeled

¼ tsp of ginger, ground

**Preparation:**

Trim off the fennel stalks and outer wilted layers. Wash and chop the fennel into bite-sized pieces. Fill the measuring cup and reserve the rest for later. Set aside.

Rinse the spinach thoroughly under cold running water and drain. Torn into small pieces and set aside.

Wash the broccoli and trim off the outer leaves. Chop into small pieces and fill the measuring cup. Reserve the rest in the refrigerator.

Peel the lemon and lime. Cut lengthwise into halves. Set aside.

Now, combine fennel, spinach, broccoli, lemon, and lime in a juicer. Process until juiced.

Transfer to a serving glass and stir in the ginger.

Add some crushed ice and serve immediately.

**Nutrition information per serving:** Kcal: 86, Protein: 10.5g, Carbs: 29.1g, Fats: 1.5g

## 36.     Blueberry Vanilla Juice

**Ingredients:**

2 cups of blueberries

1 large wedge of honeydew melon

1 small green apple, cored

1 oz of coconut water

1 tsp of vanilla extract

1 tbsp of mint, finely chopped

**Preparation:**

Place the blueberries in a large colander. Rinse well under cold running water and drain. Set aside.

Cut melon lengthwise in half. Scoop out the seeds and then wash. Cut one large wedge and peel it. Cut into small cubes and set aside.

Wash the green apple and cut lengthwise in half. Remove the core and cut into bite-sized pieces. Set aside.

Now, combine blueberries, honeydew melon, and apple in a juicer. Process until juiced.

Transfer to a serving glass and stir in the coconut water, vanilla extract, and mint. Add some crushed ice and serve immediately.

**Nutrition information per serving:** Kcal: 263, Protein: 3.7g, Carbs: 77.1g, Fats: 1.5g

## 37.    Carrot Lime Juice

**Ingredients:**

1 large carrot, sliced

1 whole lime, peeled

1 cup of mango, chunked

1 large banana, sliced

1 small Golden Delicious apple, cored

¼ tsp of cinnamon, ground

**Preparation:**

Wash and peel the carrot. Cut into thin slices and set aside.

Peel the lime and cut lengthwise in half. Set aside.

Peel the mango and cut into small chunks. Fill the measuring cup and reserve the rest in the refrigerator. Set aside.

Peel the banana and cut into slices. Set aside.

Wash the apple and cut in half. Remove the core and chop into bite-sized pieces. Set aside.

Now, combine carrot, lime, mango, banana, and apple in a juicer and process until juiced. Transfer to a serving glass and stir in the cinnamon.

Add some ice and serve immediately.

**Nutrition information per serving:** Kcal: 290, Protein: 4.1g, Carbs: 83.9g, Fats: 1.5g

# MEALS

## 1.  Ginger Cookies

**Ingredients:**

9 oz. of all-purpose flour

2 tsp of ginger, ground

½ tsp of salt

¼ tsp of cinnamon

5 oz. of butter

1 cup of honey

1 large egg

3 tbsp. of honey

**Preparation:**

Preheat the oven to 350°F.

Combine flour, ginger, salt, and cinnamon in a large mixing bowl. Stir well to combine. Set aside

Whisk the egg, butter, and honey. Now, combine both mixtures together and stir all well.

Meanwhile, line some baking paper in a large baking sheet.

Using your hands, form cookie shapes and place into a baking sheet. Bake for 10 minutes and remove from the oven to cool.

You can serve your cookies with some homemade fruit jam, or simply with a glass of milk.

Enjoy!

**Nutritional information per serving:** Kcal: 123, Protein: 0.9g, Carbs: 19.7g, Fats: 4.2g

## 2. Cinnamon Muffins

**Ingredients:**

1 cup of all-purpose flour

¼ cup of honey

1 tsp of yeast

1 tbsp. of butter, melted

2 cups of skim milk

1 tsp od salt

1 tsp of cinnamon, ground

For topping:

2 tbsp. of almond, roughly chopped

1 tbsp. of butter

1 tbsp. of honey

1 tsp of cinnamon

**Preparation:**

Combine dry ingredients in a large bowl and mix well. Now gently stir in 1 tablespoon of melted butter and milk, until the dough forms a ball. You can add some more milk to get the right consistency. Mix well for a few minutes, using your hands or an electric mixer. The dough will become very sticky.

Now add some more flour (2 tablespoons should be enough) to get a nice and smooth mixture. Cover and let it rise for about 15 minutes.

Meanwhile, preheat the oven to 350°F. Use a muffin molds to shape your muffins. Bake for about 20 minutes, until nice gold brown color. Remove from the oven to cool.

Now, combine all topping ingredients in a large skillet over a medium-high temperature. Stir and cook until it all combines, or butter melts. Pour over the topping over muffins and refrigerate for 10 minutes.

Serve!

**Nutritional information per serving:** Kcal: 145, Protein: 5.2g, Carbs: 28.4g, Fats: 10.2g

### 3.    Avocado Ziti Pesto

**Ingredients:**

10 oz. of ziti pasta,

2 medium-sized avocados, peeled, pit removed, and chopped

1 tsp of fresh basil, finely chopped

1 tsp of pine nuts, chopped (or any other that you have on hand)

½ cup of olive oil

1 tsp of salt

1 tsp of black pepper, ground

1 tbsp. of lemon juice

1 tsp of lemon zest

**Preparation:**

Follow the instructions on the package to cook ziti. Remove after cooking and transfer to serving plate.

Meanwhile, combine basil, pine nuts, avocados, lemon juice, and olive oil in large mixing bowl. Sprinkle with some salt and pepper and stir well to combine. Set the pesto aside.

Pour pesto over the ziti and season with lemon zest on top.

Enjoy!

**Nutritional information per serving:** Kcal: 447, Protein: 9.8g, Carbs: 48.2g, Fats: 23.1g

## 4.    Beets with Mint Sauce

**Ingredients:**

2 lb. of beets, trimmed and sliced

1 tbsp. of olive oil

**For dressing:**

¼ cup of mint leaves, finely chopped

1 tbsp. of lemon juice

1 tsp of honey

½ tsp of salt

**Preparation:**

Preheat the oven to 400°F.

Wrap beet slices in a greased aluminum foil and place them into the oven. Bake beets for 1 hour, or until soften. Remove from the heat and leave it while to cool.

Meanwhile, combine the dressing ingredients in a mixing bowl and whisk well the mixture.

Transfer beets to the serving plate and drizzle with dressing. Sprinkle with some extra pinch of salt and garnish with some fresh mint leaves.

**Nutritional information per serving:** Kcal: 82, Protein: 0.2g, Carbs: 2.6g, Fats: 5.1g

## 5.    Warm Chicken Bowl

**Ingredients:**

1 ½ lb. of fire roasted tomatoes, diced

12 chicken thighs, boneless and skinless

1 tbsp. of dried basil, ground

8 oz. of milk, full fat

½ tsp of salt

½ tsp of black pepper, ground

7 oz. of tomato paste

3 celery stalks, chopped

3 medium-sized carrots, chopped

2 tbsp. of olive oil

1 finely chopped onion

4 garlic cloves, minced

½ container of mushrooms

**Preparation:**

Preheat olive oil in a frying pan over medium-high temperature. Add the celery, onions and carrots and fry for 5 to 10 minutes.

Transfer to the skillet and add tomato paste, basil, garlic, mushrooms and seasoning. Keep stirring the vegetables till they are completely covered by tomato sauce. At the same time, cut the chicken into small cubes to make it easier to eat.

Put the chicken in the skillet, pour the olive oil over it and throw in the tomatoes. Stir the chicken in to ensure the ingredients and vegetables are properly mixed with it. Turn the heat to low and cook for about 30 minutes.

The vegetables and chicken should be cooked completely before you turn the heat off.

Serve

**Nutritional information per serving:** Kcal: 504, Protein: 36.3g, Carbs: 72.4g, Fats: 6.8g

## 6.    Autumn Soup

**Ingredients:**

3 medium-sized sweet potatoes, chopped

1 tsp of salt

2 sliced fennel bulbs

15 oz. of pureed pumpkin

1 large onion sliced

1 tbsp. of olive oil

½ tsp of pumpkin pie spice

50 oz. boiling water

**Preparation:**

Heat up 1 tablespoon of oil in a crock pot over a medium-high temperature.

Now, turn the heat to low and add onion and fennel bulbs. Cover with a lid and continue to cook until caramelized.

Add the rest of the ingredients to the pot and continue cooking till the sweet potatoes are sour. Cook on low heat to get the best possible result. After the process is completed, blend the soup until it is smooth and then add salt to taste.

Enjoy!

**Nutritional information per serving:** Kcal: 230, Protein: 1.3g, Carbs: 32.6g, Fats: 12.3g

## 7.    Spanish Chicken

**Ingredients:**

6 chicken thighs, skinless

½ cauliflower head, chopped

1 tsp of salt

1 can of tomatoes, chopped

½ lb. of Brussels sprouts

1 medium-sized chorizo sausage

3 medium-sized zucchinis, peeled and sliced

2 tbsp. of vegetable oil

**Preparation:**

Take a frying pan and add some oil. Fry the chicken thighs, removing the skin if you want, until they turn golden brown. Remove the thighs from the frying pan and move to a large pot. Next, chop the sausage and fry for around 3 minutes. After frying, put it in the pot as well.

Slice the zucchinis and break the cauliflower into small florets and put them in the pot as well. Also, add the Brussels sprouts to the pot. Add salt and then pour the chopped tomatoes over the ingredients. Set the heat to low and cook for about an hour. Serve with a side of baby corn.

**Nutritional information per serving:** Kcal: 431, Protein: 27.7g, Carbs: 38.4g, Fats: 13.2g

## 8.    White Mushrooms Beef Tips

**Ingredients:**

2 pounds of grass-fed beef stew meat, cubed

Salt and ground pepper, to taste

2 tablespoons of olive oil

2 cups of fresh white mushrooms

2 cups of beef stock

½ white onion, chopped

1 tablespoon minced garlic

**Preparation:**

Season the beef with salt and pepper and toss to coat it evenly with spices.

In a stew pot over medium-high heat, add the oil and brown the beef evenly on all sides. Stir in the garlic and onions, sauté for 2 minutes and add the mushrooms.

Add the oil in the inner pot, press the sauté button and adjust to brown mode. Season beef with salt and pepper and brown evenly on all sides in the inner pot. Stir in the onions and garlic and sauté for about 1 minute and then add the mushrooms and the stock. Cover with lid, bring it to a boil and reduce to low heat. Simmer for about 30 minutes or until the meat is tender and cooked through.

Adjust the seasoning and transfer into a serving bowl. Serve immediately.

**Nutritional information per serving:** Kcal: 235, Protein: 28.8g, Carbs: 18.4g, Fats: 7.2g

## 9.    Turkey in Orange Sauce

**Ingredients:**

2 tbsp. of clarified butter

1 lb. of turkey breast slices

1 tsp of salt

1 tsp of black pepper, ground

1 cup of chicken stock

2 tablespoons of butter

1 tsp of honey

2 tsp of orange zest

2 tbsp. of fresh orange, juiced

1 tsp of Cayenne pepper, ground

**Preparation:**

Season the slices of turkey evenly with salt and pepper on both sides.

Add the butter into the pan and apply medium-high heat. When the butter melts, brown the turkey meat on both sides and transfer into a plate. Set aside.

Add more butter, orange zest, orange juice, cayenne and the stock in the same pan and cook until it reaches to a simmer. Return the turkey meat in the pan and baste with sauce.

Cover with lid, bring it to a boil and reduce heat to low. Simmer for 45 to 60 minutes or until the meat is tender and cooked through. If the sauce is not yet thick, cook further without the lid until the desired consistency is achieved.

Transfer the turkey meat into a serving platter, drizzle over with sauce and serve immediately.

**Nutritional information per serving:** Kcal: 125, Protein: 13.6g, Carbs: 17.3g, Fats: 8.2g

## 10.    Thai Beef Curry with Lime

### Ingredients:

2 lb. of beef chuck steak, sliced into thin strips

2 tbsp. of olive oil

2 tbsp. lime leaves, thinly sliced

1 cup of milk, unsweetened

½ cup beef stock or water (optional)

3 tsp of sugar

1 tsp of salt

1 tsp of black pepper, ground

¼ cup of Panang curry paste

### Preparation:

Preheat one tablespoon of olive oil in a stew pot over a medium-high temperature. Briefly add one tablespoon of lime leaves.

Add in the curry paste, reduce temperature to low and cook for about 3 minutes or until aromatic.

Add the meat and cook for 5 minutes while stirring occasionally.

Stir in the sugar, pour in the stock, and milk. Briefly stir to evenly distribute the ingredients and cover with lid. Bring it to a boil and reduce heat to low. Simmer for 30 to 35 minutes or until the beef is tender and cooked through.

Adjust taste and cook further to adjust the consistency of sauce.

Portion the beef curry into individual serving bowls or transfer into a serving bowl and serve immediately.

**Nutritional information per serving:** Kcal: 425, Protein: 21.2g, Carbs: 18.9g, Fats: 23.2g

## 11.  Ground Cumin Tuna Steaks


**Ingredients:**

¼ cup of chopped fresh coriander leaves

2 garlic cloves, minced

2 tbsp. of lemon juice

½ cup of olive oil

4 tuna steaks

½ tsp of smoked paprika

½ tsp of cumin, ground

½ tsp of chili powder

¼ cup of fresh mint

**Preparation:**

Add the coriander, garlic, paprika, cumin, chili powder and lemon juice in a food processor and pulse to combine. Gradually add in the oil and pulse the ingredients until a smooth mixture is achieved.

Transfer the mixture into a bowl, add the fish and gently toss to coat the fish evenly with sauce. Chill for at least 2 hours to allow the flavors to penetrate into the fish.

Remove the fish from the chiller and preheat the gas/charcoal grill. Lightly brush the grid with oil, place the fish and grill for about 3 to 4 minutes on each side.

Remove the fish from the grill, transfer on a serving plate and serve with fresh mint leaves.

**Nutritional information per serving:** Kcal: 187, Protein: 29.2g, Carbs: 3.4g, Fats: 4.2g

## 12.    Green Bean Burritos

**Ingredients:**

1 cup of green beans, pre-cooked

1 lb. of lean ground beef

1 cup of cottage cheese, crumbled

½ cup of medium-sized onions, finely chopped

1 tsp of red pepper, ground

1 tsp of chili powder

6 whole grain tortillas

**Preparation:**

Cook up the meat and rinse it. Chop it into bite size pieces and put it back in the pan. Add ground red pepper, chili powder and onions. Stir well for 15 minutes. Remove from the heat.

Combine cottage cheese with green beans in a blender. Mix well for 30 seconds. Add the cheese mixture to the meat. Divide this mixture into 6 equal pieces and spread over tortillas. Wrap and serve.

**Nutritional information per serving:** Kcal: 248, Protein: 2.4g, Carbs: 7.4g, Fats: 2.1g

## 13.    Egg and Avocado Puree

**Ingredients:**

4 free-range eggs

1 cup of skim milk

½ avocado, peeled, pit removed, chopped

1 tsp of salt

**Preparation:**

Gently place two eggs in a pot of boiling water. Cook for 10 minutes. Rinse and drain. Cool for a while and peel. You can add one teaspoon of baking soda in a boiling water. This will make the peeling process much easier. Cut the eggs into bite-sized pieces and refrigerate for about 30 minutes.

Place avocado chops and eggs into the blender. Season with salt to taste. Add milk and blend for 30 seconds or until smooth. This puree should be eaten right away.

**Nutritional information per serving:** Kcal: 221, Protein: 9.8g, Carbs: 9.5g, Fats: 18.2g

## 14.    Creamy Strawberry Salad

**Ingredients:**

½ cup of walnuts, ground

2 cups of fresh strawberries, chopped

1 tbsp. of strawberry syrup

2 tbsp. of whipping cream

1 tbsp. of brown sugar

**Preparation:**

Wash and cut the strawberries into small pieces. Mix with ground walnuts in a bowl. In a separate bowl, combine strawberry syrup, nonfat cream and brown sugar. Beat well with a fork and use to top the salad.

**Nutritional information per serving:** Kcal: 223, Protein: 12.3g, Carbs: 10.2g, Fats: 4.8g

## 15.    Ginger Eggs

**Ingredients:**

3 free-range eggs

2 tbsp. of olive oil

1 tsp of fresh ginger, grated

¼ tsp of black pepper, ground

¼ tsp of sea salt

**Preparation:**

Beat the eggs with a fork. Add ginger and pepper. Mix well and fry in olive oil for few minutes. Serve warm. Season with sea salt.

**Nutritional information per serving:** Kcal: 102, Protein: 13.7g, Carbs: 9.5g, Fats: 5.6g

## 16.    Buckwheat Chia Bread

**Ingredients:**

3 cups of buckwheat flour

3 egg whites

1 cup of chia seeds, minced

1 tsp of salt

½ pack of dry yeast

Warm water

**Preparation:**

Mix flour, eggs and chia seeds with salt and yeast. Add warm water and stir until smooth dough. Let it stand in a warm place for about 30-40 minutes.

Spread some flour on a working surface. This will prevent the dough from sticking. Now shape the bread using your hands. I always like to shape round breads, but this is not necessary.

Sprinkle with cold water and bake in preheated oven, at 350 degrees for about 40 minutes.

**Nutritional information per serving:** Kcal: 131, Protein: 6.8g, Carbs: 16.3g, Fats: 4.2g

## 17.    Warm Bean Salad

**Ingredients:**

14oz of beans, pre-cooked

7oz sweet corn

1 tsp of chili powder

1 tbsp. of chopped parsley

3 tbsp. of oil

1 medium-sized onion, peeled and chopped

**Preparation:**

Heat up the oil over a medium temperature. Stir-fry the onion for a couple of minutes. Add chili pepper and about two tablespoons of water and continue to cook for ten more minutes.

Now add the beans, corn, and about ¼ cup of water. Bring it to a boil and cook for another ten minutes. Remove from the heat and transfer to a bowl.

Add chopped parsley and toss to combine. Serve.

**Nutritional information per serving:** Kcal: 121 Protein: 36g, Carbs: 30.8g, Fats: 14g

## 18.    Cottage Cheese Chia Pate

**Ingredients:**

½ cup of chia seeds powder

¼ cup of chia seeds

½ cup of cottage cheese, crumbled

¼ cup of parsley, finely chopped

¼ cup of skim milk

1 tbsp. of mustard

¼ tsp of salt

**Preparation:**

Combine parsley and mustard in a mixing bowl and set aside.

Meanwhile, combine cottage cheese with milk, salt, chia seeds powder, and chia seeds. Mix well, add parsley and mustard mixture. Allow it to stand in the refrigerator for about an hour before serving

**Nutritional information per serving:** Kcal: 131, Protein: 14.8g, Carbs: 10.3g, Fats: 7.4g

## 19.    Sunflower Chicken Salad

**Ingredients:**

3 chicken breast, skinless and boneless, halved

1 cup of Iceberg lettuce, torn

5 cherry tomatoes, halved

2 tbsp. of sour cream

1 tbsp. of olive oil

1 tsp of fresh parsley, chopped

1 tbsp. of sunflower oil

1 tsp of chili pepper, ground

1 tbsp. of lemon juice

1 tsp of salt

**Preparation:**

Cut the chicken breast halves into bite-sized pieces. Mix the sunflower oil, chopped parsley, minced chili pepper, and lemon juice to make a marinade. Put the chicken cubes on a baking sheet, sprinkle with chili marinade and bake at 350 degrees for about 30 minutes. Remove from the oven.

Meanwhile, mix cherry tomatoes with chopped lettuce and low fat cream. Add chicken cubes and season with salt and olive oil.

Toss to combine and serve.

**Nutritional information per serving:** Kcal: 282, Protein: 29.4g, Carbs: 9.8g, Fats: 12.3g

## 20.    Creamy Green Beans

**Ingredients:**

1 cup of green beans, pre-cooked

1 medium-sized tomato, chopped

1 ½ cup of cottage cheese

1 tsp of garlic sauce

1 tbsp. of flaxseed oil

1 tsp of salt

1 tsp of black pepper, ground

**Preparation:**

You should buy pre-cooked beans for this one as it will save you some time. If, however, you choose to cook beans yourself, soak them overnight, rinse, and drain before cooking. Place in a deep pot and add enough water to cover.

Cook for 35-40 minutes over medium-high heat. Drain and chill for a while.

Meanwhile, finely chop tomato and place in a bowl. Add other ingredients and toss well to combine. Season with salt and pepper. Serve cold.

**Nutritional information per serving:** Kcal: 192, Protein: 11.3g, Carbs: 20.5g, Fats: 8.7g

## 21.    Baby Spinach and Egg Salad

### Ingredients:

4 large eggs, boiled

1 medium-sized carrot, grated

1 cup of baby spinach, chopped

1 tbsp. of fresh ginger, grated

1 tbsp. of lemon juice

1 tbsp. of olive oil

1 tsp of turmeric, grated

1 tsp of salt

### Preparation:

Boil the eggs for about 10-12 minutes, remove from heat, peel and cut into small cubes. Place in a large bowl and combine with spinach, grated carrot, and ginger.

Sprinkle with lemon juice, and season with olive oil, turmeric, and salt. Serve cold.

**Nutritional information per serving:** Kcal: 97, Protein: 13.3g, Carbs: 4.5g, Fats: 3.5g

## 22.    Red Cabbage with Feta

### Ingredients:

1 cup of red cabbage, grated

½ cup of carrots, grated

½ cup of beetroot, grated

1 cup of feta cheese

3 tbsp. of almonds, minced

1 tbsp. of almond extract

1 tbsp. of vegetable oil

1 tsp of salt

### Preparation:

Mix the vegetables in a large bowl. Add feta cheese, minced almonds and almond extract. Season with almond oil and salt.

You can add some lemon juice or vinegar, but that is optional.

**Nutritional information per serving:** Kcal: 98, Protein: 5.8g, Carbs: 7.2g, Fats: 8.5g

## 23.    Mediterranean Fish Balls

**Ingredients:**

1½ lbs. white fish, boneless

1 tsp of black pepper, freshly ground

½ lb. of shrimps

½ lemon juice

1½ cup of almond flour

2 tbsp. of tartar sauce

½ cup water

3 tbsp. of fresh parsley, finely chopped

3 large eggs

1 tsp of salt

Cooking spray

**Preparation:**

Use a food processor to make a paste combining 2 eggs, ½ cup almond flour, shrimps, white fish, parsley, and lemon juice, blending till the paste is smooth. Take a bowl, pour some water and break an egg into it. Whisk the two and create a mixture. In a separate bowl, put the remaining almond flour and add salt and pepper to it.

Take a larger bowl and mix the contents of all three bowls. Then, make small balls out of the batter you have created. Put the balls in the skillet and fry for about 15 minutes. Enjoy with tartar sauce.

**Nutritional information per serving:** Kcal: 54, Protein: 5.2g, Carbs: 4.7g, Fats: 2.5g

## 24.  Butter Shrimps

**Ingredients:**

2 lbs. of large shrimps, peeled and deveined

2 tbsp. lemon juice

1 tsp Cayenne pepper, ground

½ tsp of black pepper, ground

1 tsp of sea salt

4 garlic cloves, minced

3 tbsp. of butter

2 tbsp. of fresh parsley, chopped

2 tbsp. of cooking fat

**Preparation:**

Preheat a large skillet over a medium-high temperature. Add some butter, and cook until melts.

Now, add in the shrimps. Fry the shrimps till almost opaque in appearance.

Add the rest of the ingredients to the skillet. Reduce the heat to low and cook for 30 minutes more.

**Nutritional information per serving:** Kcal: 104, Protein: 19.6g, Carbs: 4.8g, Fats: 11.7g

## 25.    Parsley with Nuts & Dates Salad

**Ingredients:**

2 cups of Italian parsley, roughly chopped

¼ cup of almonds, halved

½ cup of dates, pit removed and halved

2 tbsp. of balsamic vinegar

2 tbsp. of olive oil

½ tsp of salt

½ tsp of black pepper, ground

**Preparation:**

Combine the oil, vinegar, salt, and pepper in a small mixing bowl. Whisk well and set aside.

In large salad bowl, combine parsley, almonds, and dates. Toss well and drizzle with dressing.

Refrigerate for 30 minutes before serving.

**Nutritional information per serving:** Kcal: 58, Protein: 5.2g, Carbs: 10.6g, Fats: 8.7g

## 26.  Soft Cumin Pork Chops

**Ingredients:**

4 lbs. of loin pork chops, trimmed

1 tbsp. of brown sugar

1 tsp of salt

1 tsp of chili pepper, ground

**For dressing:**

1 tsp of cumin, ground

1 tsp of Dijon mustard

½ tsp of smoked paprika, ground

½ tsp of black pepper, ground

1 tbsp. of olive oil

**Preparation:**

Preheat the oil in a large frying skillet over a medium-high temperature.

Meanwhile, combine dressing ingredients in a mixing bowl and set aside.

Place the pork chops into the pan and cook for about 10 minutes from both sides, or until doneness. Reduce the heat to low and cook for 5 minutes more. Remove from the heat and transfer the meat to the serving plate.

Top the meat with dressing.

Serve with some fresh sliced tomatoes. This is, however, optional.

**Nutritional information per serving:** Kcal: 165, Protein: 24.6g, Carbs: 3.5g, Fats: 12.4g

## 27.    No Bake Coconut Cookies

**Ingredients:**

2 tbsp. of walnuts, roughly chopped

½ small coconut, grated

1 tbsp. of Goji berries

1 cup of coconut milk

1tsp of lemon zest

½ tsp of vanilla extract

½ tsp of sugar

1 tsp of cocoa, raw

½ tsp of chili, ground

**Preparation:**

Combine chili, lemon zest, vanilla extract and coconut milk in a medium deep pot. Cook for about 10 to 15 minutes on a low temperature. Leave it to cool for a while.

Meanwhile, combine walnuts, coconut chops, berries and half cup of water in a food processor. Blend until smooth and transfer to the pot. Give it a final stir to combine.

Use muffin molds to shape cookies. Top with cocoa or grated chocolate and refrigerate for 3 hours before serving.

**Nutritional information per serving:** Kcal: 135, Protein: 3.2g, Carbs: 10.2g, Fats: 9.4g

## 28.    Parsley Toast

**Ingredients:**

4 slices of grain bread, whole

½ cup of Mozzarella cheese, crumbled

½ cup of parsley, finely chopped

2 tbsp. of extra virgin olive oil

1 tsp of black pepper, ground

1 tsp of basil, ground

**Preparation:**

Combine cheese, parsley, and pepper in mixing bowl. Beat well with a fork and set aside.

Spread the olive oil onto bread slices using a kitchen brush. Place the bread slices in the toaster and set for 2 minutes, or medium toasted.

Spread mixture over the bread slices. Sprinkle with extra teaspoon of ground basil. Eat immediately while warm and crunchy.

You can add a few tomato slices, but this is optional.

Enjoy!

**Nutritional information per serving:** Kcal: 145, Protein: 8.8g, Carbs: 15.7g, Fats: 5.5g

## 29.  Overnight Pomegranate Oatmeal

**Ingredients:**

1 cup of oatmeal

½ cup of dried plums, chopped

1 cup of skim milk

1 tbsp. of flaxseed

1 tbsp. of honey

1 tbsp. of pomegranate seeds

1 tbsp. of chia seeds

1 tsp of vanilla extract

¼ cup of pomegranate juice

**Preparation:**

First, combine oatmeal, plums, flaxseed, and vanilla extract in a large mixing bowl. Add milk, honey, pomegranate juice, and stir all well to combine. Top with chia seeds and refrigerate overnight.

**Nutritional information per serving:** Kcal: 310, Protein: 12.4g, Carbs: 41.2g, Fats: 9.3g

## 30.　　Shrimp Stew with Fire Roasted Tomatoes

**Ingredients:**

1 cup of fire roasted tomatoes

1 cup of frozen shrimp mix

1 tbsp. of dry basil

4 cups fish stock

3 tbsp. of tomato paste

3 pieces' celery stalks, chopped

3 medium-sized carrots, chopped

2 tbsp. of olive oil

1 medium-sized onion, finely chopped

4 garlic cloves, crushed

½ cup of button mushrooms

**Preparation:**

Heat up the olive oil in a frying pan, over a medium temperature. Add chopped celery, onions, and carrots. Stir well and fry for about 10 minutes.

Remove from the heat and transfer to a deep pot. Add the remaining ingredients and cook for about an hour over a medium temperature. "

**Nutritional information per serving:** Kcal: 303, Protein: 34.8g, Carbs: 7.4g, Fats: 15.3g

## 31.    Avocado Pancakes

**Ingredients:**

1 cup of skim milk

1 free-range egg

1 cup of all-purpose flour

½ tsp of salt

1 medium-sized avocado, peeled and pit removed, chopped

½ tbsp. of brown sugar

2 tbsp. of oil for frying

1 tsp of sugar powder

1 tsp of baking powder

**Preparation:**

Preheat the oil in a frying skillet over a medium-high temperature.

Meanwhile, combine flour, baking powder, and salt in large mixing bowl. Stir well and add milk and egg.

Stir all well until you get smooth dough mixture. Spoon in mixture into the skillet, and fry until gold brown on both sides. Baked pancakes remove to cool.

Put avocado chops into the food processor. Sprinkle with brown sugar and blend until smooth.

Spread avocado mixture on the pancakes and sprinkle with some sugar powder for decoration.

Serve immediately.

**Nutritional information per serving:** Kcal: 198, Protein: 7.6g, Carbs: 12.5g, Fats: 12.3g

## 32.    Creamy White Chili

**Ingredients:**

1 pound of chicken breast, boneless and skinless, cut into ½ inch thick cubes

1 medium-sized onion, peeled and sliced

2 cans of white beans, cooked

1 can of chicken broth

2 cans of green chilies, chopped

3 tbsp. of olive oil

Salt and pepper to taste

1 tsp of oregano, dry

1 tsp of cumin, ground

1 cup of sour cream

½ cup of heavy whipping cream

**Preparation:**

Heat up the olive oil over a medium-high temperature. Add the sliced onions and garlic. Stir-fry for about a minute and add the chicken cubes. Reduce the heat to medium and cook for about 15 minutes.

Add other ingredients, except the sour cream and heavy whipping cream. Mix well and bring it to a boil. Reduce the heat to low, cover and cook for about 30 minutes.

Top with sour cream and heavy whipping cream. Serve warm.

**Nutritional information per serving:** Kcal: 206 Protein: 45.4g, Carbs: 49g, Fats: 17g

## 33.    Green Tea Smoothie

**Ingredients:**

3 tbsp. of green tea, minced

1 cup of grapes, white

½ cup of kale, finely chopped

1 tbsp. of honey

½ tsp of fresh mint, ground

1 cup of water

**Preparation:**

Combine all ingredients in a blender. Blend until smooth and transfer into the smoothie glasses. Refrigerate 30 minutes before serving.

Serve immediately with some ice cubes.

**Nutritional information per serving:** Kcal: 301 Protein: 4.8g, Carbs: 55.4g, Fats: 2.1g

## 34.   Thick Chicken Soup

**Ingredients:**

1 pound of chicken meat, boneless and skinless

1 can of white beans

¼ jalapeno pepper, chopped

1 small onion, peeled and finely chopped

2 garlic cloves, crushed

3 tbsp. of vegetable oil

1 tsp of salt

1 tsp of black pepper, ground

2 cups of chicken broth

½ tsp of chili powder

¼ cup of lime juice

½ tsp of cumin, ground

½ tsp of coriander, ground

**Preparation:**

Rinse and drain the beans. Mash half of the beans with a fork and set aside.

Heat up the oil in a large frying skillet, over a medium temperature. Add garlic, onions and peppers. Stir-fry for several minutes.

Now, add the spices and continue to fry for another minute or two.

Add the beans, chicken meat, chicken broth and lime juice. Bring it to a boil and cook for about 20 minutes.

Add the cilantro and cook for five more minutes. Remove from the heat and let it cool.

Serve!

**Nutritional information per serving:** Kcal: 118, Protein: 36g, Carbs: 31.8g, Fats: 16g

## 35.    Brussels Sprouts in Tomato Sauce

**Ingredients:**

3 lbs. of oxtail, pre – cooked and boneless

1 ½ lb. of Brussel sprouts, pre – cooked and drained

1 large red onion

4 garlic cloves

1 tbsp. of chili powder

1 large tomato, blended

3 bay leaves

½ cup of fresh parsley, minced

4 cups of water

1 tbsp. of olive oil

**Preparation:**

Pour 6 glasses of water into the pressure pot and add the oxtail. Add 1 tbsp. of olive oil and cook for 10 minutes.

Add all vegetables and spices. Water level must cover all ingredients. Add until it is enough. Cook for 45 minutes.

Blend the tomato and transfer mixture into the pressure pot. Cook for more 20 minutes.

**Nutritional information per serving:** Kcal: 219, Protein: 48.3g, Carbs: 51.4g Fats: 29g

## 36.　　Creamy Squid

### Ingredients:

1 lb. of fresh squid, without the heads

1 cup of cottage cheese

½ cup of Feta cheese

¼ cup of fresh celery, finely chopped"

3 tbsp. of olive oil

1 tsp chili pepper, ground

### Preparation:

Wash and clean the squid. Pat dry and set aside.

Combine the cottage cheese with Feta cheese, and chopped celery. Mix well and use 1 tbsp. of this mixture to fill each squid.

Heat up the olive oil in a large skillet over medium-high temperature. Fry the squid on each side for several minutes. Remove from the skillet and allow it to cool for about 15 minutes.

Sprinkle with ground chili pepper and serve.

**Nutritional information per serving:** Kcal: 232, Protein: 24.2g, Carbs: 9.1g, Fats: 10.5g

## 37.    Warm Carrot Soup

**Ingredients:**

5 large carrots, peeled and sliced

2 tbsp. of olive oil

1 cup of cooking cream

2 cups of water

¼ tsp of salt

**Preparation:**

Heat up the olive oil over a medium temperature. Peel and slice the carrots. Fry for about 15 minutes, stirring constantly.

Reduce the heat, add cooking cream, salt and water. Cook for about 10 minutes.

**Nutritional information per serving**: Kcal: 115, Protein: 5.8g, Carbs: 16.3g, Fats: 3.4g

## 38.    Warm Vanilla Pudding

**Ingredients:**

2 cups of milk

½ cup of sugar

2 tbsp. of vanilla extract

3 tbsp. of cornstarch

1 tbsp. of butter

**Preparation:**

In a medium-sized saucepan, heat the milk until it starts to boil. Meanwhile, combine the sugar with cornstarch and mix well. Pour the mixture into hot milk and mix well. Reduce the heat to minimum and cook until the mixture thickens. Stir in one tablespoon of butter and vanilla extract. Pour into serving glasses and cool well.

Top with chocolate ice cream and some chocolate dessert topping.

**Nutritional information per serving**: Kcal: 145, Protein: 3.1g, Carbs: 25.2g, Fats: 4.5g

## 39.    Roasted Lamb Chops

**Ingredients:**

5 lamb loin chops, 1 ½ inch thick sliced

1 cup of vegetable oil

3 garlic cloves, crushed

1 tbsp. of fresh thyme leaves, crushed

1 tbsp. of fresh rosemary, crushed

1 tbsp. of red pepper, ground

1 tsp sea salt

**Preparation:**

Combine the oil with crushed garlic cloves, fresh thyme leaves, fresh rosemary, red pepper, and salt. Mix well in a large bowl. Add lamb loin chops and turn to coat. Let it stand in the refrigerator for about 2 hours.

Preheat the oven to 350°F.

Place the lamb chops in a large, ovenproof skillet. Add 4 tablespoons of the marinade and reduce the heat to 300°F. Cook for about 15 minutes and remove from the oven.

Now add 4 tablespoons more marinade, turn over the chops, and cook for 15 more minutes.

Remove from the oven and serve with fresh vegetables. Enjoy!

**Nutritional information per serving**: Kcal: 250, Protein: 26.2g, Carbs: 14.7g, Fats: 5.6g

## 40.    Fresh Lime Salad

**Ingredients:**

1 cup of lamb's lettuce, chopped

1 large onion, sliced

6-7 medium-sized cherry tomatoes

½ cup of black olives

6-7 medium radishes

½ medium fresh lime, sliced

1 tbsp. of fresh lime juice

2 tbsp. extra virgin olive oil

½ tsp of salt

**Preparation:**

Wash and clean the vegetables. Slice the onions and mix with other vegetables in a large bowl.

Add fresh lime juice, olive oil, and salt. Mix well again. Decorate with lime slices. Enjoy!

**Nutritional information per serving**: Kcal: 163, Protein: 3.2g, Carbs: 8.7g, Fats: 512.9g

## 41.  Wild Salmon Wraps

**Ingredients:**

1lb of wild salmon, minced

1 tbsp. of mixed vegetable seasoning

1 cup chopped onion

2 tbsp. of red pepper, ground

½ cup of tomato puree

8 large Iceberg lettuce leaves

½ cup of shredded cheddar cheese

1 tbsp.       of vegetable oil

½ cup of chicken stock

**Preparation:**

Heat up some oil in a non-stick pan over medium-high temperature. Add the salmon meat and cook for 5 minutes, stirring constantly. Stir in the vegetable seasoning, onions, bell pepper and tomato puree and cook it for 5 minutes.

Pour in the water or stock, cover with lid and bring it to a boil. Reduce the heat to low and simmer for about 20 minutes, or until the liquid has reduced in half. Remove the pan from heat and set it aside.

Prepare the lettuce leaves and place them on a work surface. Portion the meat into the 6 to 8 lettuce leaves. Add cheddar cheese and wrap.

**Nutritional information per serving**: Kcal: 250, Protein: 21.2g, Carbs: 0.5g, Fats: 18.2g

## 42.    Mushrooms with Tomato Sauce

### Ingredients:

1 cup of button mushrooms

1 large tomato, peeled and chopped

3 tbsp. of olive oil

1 tbsp. of parsley, finely chopped

1 tsp of salt

½ tsp of black pepper, ground

### Preparation:

Preheat the oven to 400°F.

Preheat the oil in a frying skillet over a medium-high temperature. Pour in tomato mixture and add one cup of water. Reduce the heat to low and cook for 15 minutes until water evaporates.

Meanwhile, combine tomato, parsley, and salt into blender. Blend until smooth and set aside.

Wash and drain mushrooms and place into the large baking sheet. Spread the sauce over and sprinkle some pepper to taste.

Bake for 10-15 minutes. Remove from the oven and leave it to cool for a while.

Serve with sour cream or Greek yogurt. However, this is optional

Enjoy!

**Nutritional information per serving**: Kcal: 250, Protein: 26.2g, Carbs: 14.7g, Fats: 5.6g

## 43.    Guava Smoothie

**Ingredients:**

1 cup of guava, seeds removed, chopped

1 cup of baby spinach, finely chopped

1 banana, peeled and sliced

1 tsp of fresh ginger, grated

½ medium-sized mango, peeled and chopped

2 cups of water

**Preparation:**

Combine all ingredients in a blender. Blend until smooth and transfer to a serving glasses. Refrigerate for 30 minutes before serving.

**Nutritional information per serving:** Kcal: 242, Protein: 6.7g, Carbs: 57.4g, Fats: 1.1g

## 44.    Blue Cheese and Bean Dip

**Ingredients:**

2oz of butter

1 small onion, peeled and chopped

2 garlic cloves, crushed

8.8oz (1 can) of chili beans, pre-cooked

3.5 oz. blue cheese, grated

1 tsp of salt

½ cup of water

½ tsp of chili powder

**Preparation:**

Melt the butter over a medium temperature. Add the onions, crushed garlic, and stir-fry for several minutes, or until nice light brown color.

Add the chili beans and grated cheese. Mix well and cook until the cheese melts. Remove from the heat and chill for a while. Transfer to a blender and mix well for 30 seconds.

Add chili powder and some salt to taste. Mix well and serve.

**Nutritional information per serving:** Kcal: 71, Protein: 4.3g, Carbs: 17.5g, Fats: 9.1g

## 45.    Turkey and Veal Braid

**Ingredients:**

2 lbs. of turkey breasts, boneless and skinless

1 lb. of veal steak, boneless

¼ cup of vegetable oil

1 tsp red pepper, ground

1 tsp of sea salt

**Preparation:**

Wash and pat dry the meat. Slice the meat into ½ inch thick slices and pound each slice with a mallet. Using a sharp knife, cut the meat slices into 3 equal pieces. Secure the upper part with a toothpick, and braid.

Combine the vegetable oil with red pepper and salt. Spread this mixture over your braids using a kitchen brush. Allow it to stand for about 15 minutes.

Meanwhile, preheat the grill pan over a medium temperature. You can add 1 teaspoon of the marinade in your pan, but that is not necessary.

Fry the braids for about 10 minutes on each side, or until a nice golden color.

**Nutritional information per serving:** Kcal: 233, Protein: 29.3g, Carbs: 0.2g, Fats: 13.4g

## 46.    Stuffed Bell Pepper Salad

**Ingredients:**

3 large red bell peppers, whole

1 cup of Feta cheese, crumbled

3 egg whites

3 tbsp. sour cream

½ cup of fresh parsley, finely chopped

**Preparation:**

Wash and clean the bell peppers. Cut off the tops and remove the ribs and seeds. Rinse well. Sprinkle the inside of each bell pepper with some olive oil. Set aside.

Combine the Feta cheese, egg whites, sour cream, and fresh parsley in a bowl. Mix well. Fill the peppers with the Feta mixture.

Serve.

**Nutritional information per serving:** Kcal: 185, Protein: 11.3g, Carbs: 6.2g, Fats: 13.4g

## 47.    Creamy Mac & Cheese

**Ingredients:**

1 cup of rice macaroni

½ cup of button mushrooms, sliced

1 small tomato, peeled and chopped

¼ tsp of oregano, ground

½ tsp of brown sugar

2 tbsp. Parmesan cheese

2 tbsp. of sour cream

2 tbsp. of Feta cheese, crumbled

¼ tsp of salt

2 tbsp. of olive oil

**Preparation:**

Boil 3 cups of water in a deep pot. Remove from the heat and place the rice macaroni in it. Let it stand for several minutes. Rice macaroni will soften very quickly so be careful with this. Remove from the pot and drain. Set aside.

Preheat the olive oil over a medium temperature. Finely chop the tomato and fry for about 5 minutes stirring constantly. Add sliced mushrooms, oregano, sugar, and about 1/5 cup of water. Cook for about 10 more minutes. Remove from the heat and add macaroni. Mix well.

Melt the Feta cheese over a minimum temperature. Add sour cream and Parmesan cheese. Mix well. You can add some milk if the mixture is too thick (about 1/4 cup will be enough).

Serve macaroni with tomatoes and mushrooms and pour with cheese mixture.

**Nutritional information per serving:** Kcal: 180, Protein: 6.8g, Carbs: 22.2g, Fats: 7.3g

## 48.    Cherry Tomatoes Rice

**Ingredients:**

1 cup brown rice

6 large cherry tomatoes

1 cup button mushrooms

1 tsp dried rosemary, finely chopped

1/8 tsp of salt

3 tbsp. of olive oil

**Preparation:**

Use a package instructions to prepare the rice. Set aside.

Heat up the olive oil in a large skillet. Finely chop the tomatoes and fry for about 10 minutes stirring constantly.

Add the mushrooms and fry until all the water evaporates. Now add dry rosemary and salt.

Mix the tomato sauce with the rice and serve.

**Nutritional information per serving:** Kcal: 255, Protein: 6.1g, Carbs: 48.4g, Fats: 4.3g

## 49.    Warm Dip Tortillas

**Ingredients:**

8 tortillas

11oz of grated Gouda cheese

4 spring onions, finely chopped

5.6oz can corn

2 tbsp. of oil

For chili dip:

3 large ripe tomatoes

1 tbsp. of butter (can be replaced with olive oil)

1 tbsp. of ground chili

2 chili peppers, finely chopped

2 garlic cloves, crushed

½ tsp of dry oregano

¼ tsp of salt

1 tsp of sugar

¼ cup of white wine

## Preparation:

Heat up a grill pan over a medium-high temperature. Heat each tortilla for about one minute in a microwave. This will make a wrapping process much easier. Spread the gouda over each tortilla and add spring onions, corn and some salt. Wrap and grill each tortilla for about 1-2 minutes on each side, or until the cheese melts. Transfer to a serving platter.

## Dip:

Peel and roughly chop the tomatoes. Make sure you keep all the liquid.

Melt the butter over a medium temperature. Add the garlic and stir-fry for several minutes. Now add tomatoes, oregano, salt, sugar, ground chili and finely chopped chili peppers. Reduce the heat to low and cook until the tomatoes have softened. Add wine and cook for 10 more minutes stirring constantly. Serve with tortillas.

**Nutritional information per serving:** Kcal: 86 Protein: 4.4g, Carbs: 11.5g, Fats: 6.7g

## ADDITIONAL TITLES FROM THIS AUTHOR

70 Effective Meal Recipes to Prevent and Solve Being Overweight: Burn Fat Fast by Using Proper Dieting and Smart Nutrition

By Joe Correa CSN

48 Acne Solving Meal Recipes: The Fast and Natural Path to Fixing Your Acne Problems in Less Than 10 Days!

By Joe Correa CSN

41 Alzheimer's Preventing Meal Recipes: Reduce or Eliminate Your Alzheimer's Condition in 30 Days or Less!

By Joe Correa CSN

70 Effective Breast Cancer Meal Recipes: Prevent and Fight Breast Cancer with Smart Nutrition and Powerful Foods

By Joe Correa CSN

www.ingramcontent.com/pod-product-compliance
Lightning Source LLC
Chambersburg PA
CBHW030250030426
42336CB00009B/325